The Original Keto Diet Book 2021

Quick and Delicious Weight Loss Recipes for Everyone incl. 30 Days Diet Plan

Maria J. Marks

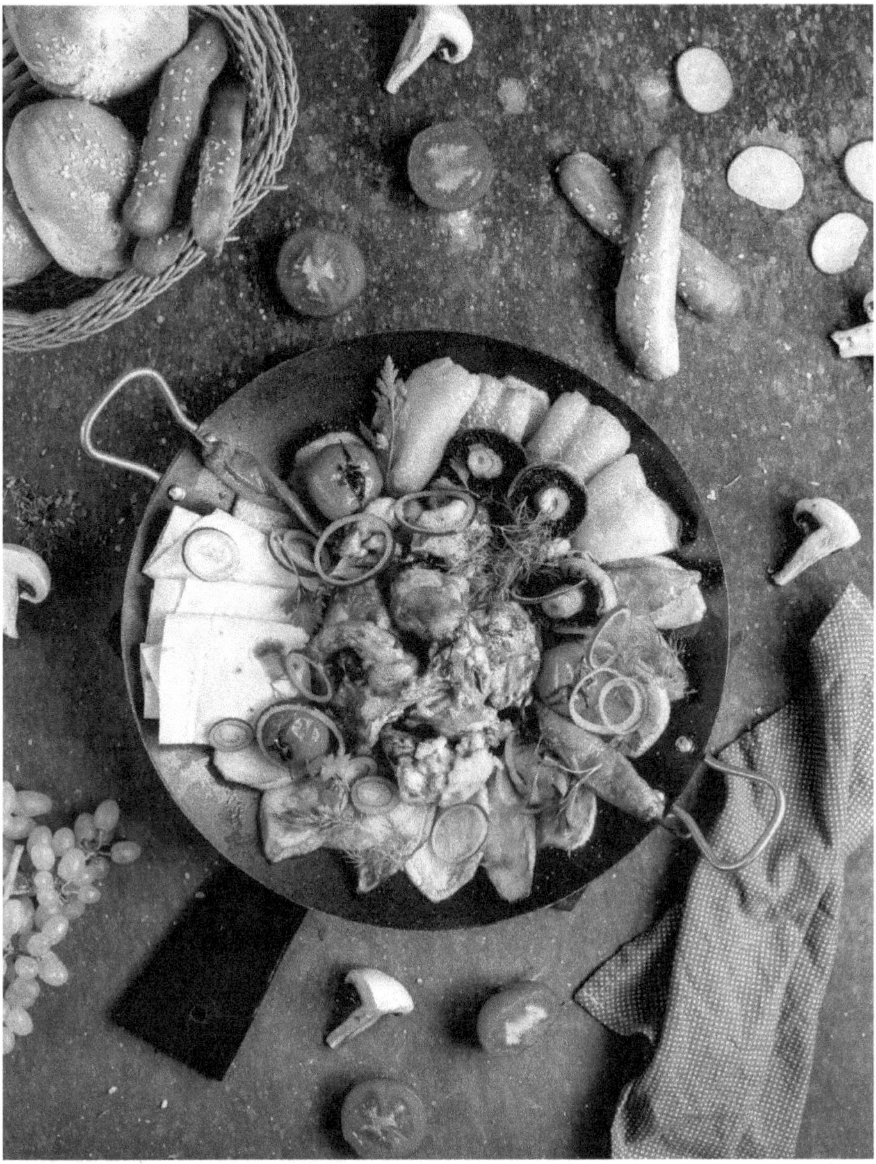

Table of Contents

Lamb Meatballs in Tomato Gravy 7

Sausage with Bell Peppers 9

Turkey Meatballs Soup 11

Shrimp with Zucchini 15

Cheesy Pork Casserole 18

Chicken Soup 22

Bacon & Avocado Soup 24

Berries & Spinach Salad 26

Chicken Burgers 27

Turkey Salad 29

Beef Stew 31

Grouper Curry 34

Chicken with Spinach 36

Broccoli Soup 39

Salmon Burgers 40

Chicken Meatballs with Guacamole 42

Chicken Chili 45

Beef & Veggie Wraps 47

Lobster Salad 50

Savory Zucchini Cake 51

Green Beans with Mushrooms 54

Steak Salad 55

Pork Stew 58

Turkey Chili 60

Steak in Mushroom Sauce 62
Stuffed Leg of Lamb 66
Cabbage Bake 69
Cheese Stuffed Turkey Burgers 72
Bacon & Tomato Salad 76
Tuna Burgers 78
Chicken Stew 80
Beef Curry 82
Lamb Curry 85
Steak with Blueberry Sauce 89
Crab Salad 92

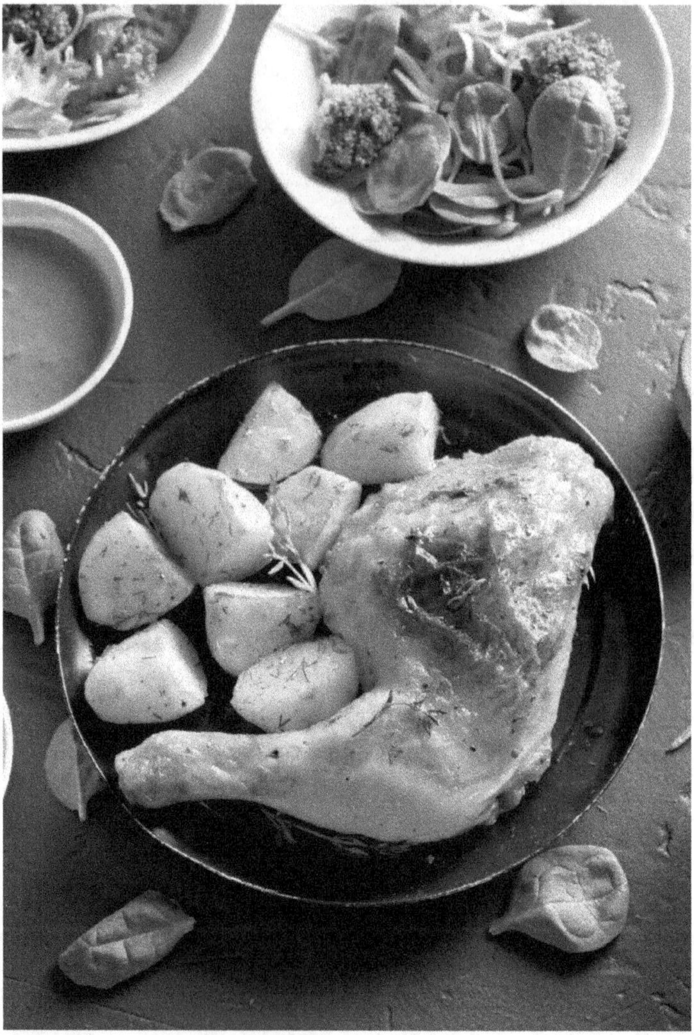

Lamb Meatballs in Tomato Gravy

Serves: 6 / Preparation time: 20 minutes / Cooking time: 35 minutes

For Meatballs

1 pound grass-fed lean ground lamb 1 tablespoon sugar-free

tomato paste

¼ cup fresh cilantro leaves, chopped 1 small yellow onion,

chopped finely

2 garlic cloves, minced ½ teaspoon ground cumin

Salt and ground black pepper, as required

For Tomato Gravy

3 tablespoons olive oil, divided 1 large yellow onions,

chopped finely

2 garlic cloves, minced ½ tablespoon fresh ginger,

minced

1 teaspoon dried thyme, crushed 1 teaspoon ground cumin

1 teaspoon cayenne pepper 3 large tomatoes, chopped

finely

Salt and ground black pepper, as required 1½ cups warm homemade

chicken broth

- For meatballs: in a large bowl, add all the ingredients and mix until

well combined.

- Make small equal sized balls from mixture and set aside.
- For gravy: in a large pan, heat 1 tablespoon of oil over medium heat

and cook the meatballs for about 4-5 minutes or until lightly browned

from all sides.

- Transfer the meatballs onto a plate.
- In the same pan, heat remaining oil over medium heat and sauté the

onion for about 4-5 minutes.

- Add the garlic, ginger, thyme and spices and sauté for about 1

minute.

- Add the tomatoes and cook for about 3-4 minutes, crushing with the back of spoon.

• Add the warm broth and bring to a boil.

• Carefully, place meatballs into the gravy and cook for about 5

minutes, without stirring.• Reduce the heat to low and cook, partially covered for about 15-20

minutes, stirring carefully 2-3 times.

• Serve hot.

• Meal Prep Tip: Transfer the meatballs mixture into a large bowl and

set aside to cool completely. Divide the mixture into 6 containers

evenly. Cover the containers and refrigerate for up to 3-4 days.

Reheat in the microwave before serving.

One Serving: Net Carbs: 5.5g; Calories: 318; Total Fat: 25.7g; Sat. Fat:

9.2g; Protein: 25.4g; Carbs: 7.5g; Fiber: 2g; Sugar: 4g

Sausage with Bell Peppers

Serves: 6 / Preparation time: 15 minutes / Cooking time:

17 minutes

1 tablespoon olive oil 8 gluten-free Italian chicken

sausages, sliced

1 large red bell pepper, seeded and sliced thinly

1 large green bell pepper, seeded and sliced thinly

1 large orange bell pepper, seeded and sliced thinly

1 teaspoon garlic powder Salt and ground black pepper,

as required

- In a large skillet, heat the oil over medium-high heat and cook

sausage for about 8-10 minutes.

- Transfer the sausage slices into a large bowl and set aside.

- In the same skillet, add the bell peppers and garlic powder and sauté

for about 3-5 minutes.

- Stir in the sausage, salt and black pepper and cook for about 1-2

minutes.

- Serve hot.

- Meal Prep Tip: Remove the sausage from heat and set

aside to cool

completely. In 4 containers, divide sausage mixture evenly and

refrigerate for about 1 day. Reheat in microwave before serving.

One Serving: Net Carbs: 3.2g; Calories: 166; Total Fat: 10.5gg; Sat. Fat:

1.7g; Protein: 12.7g; Carbs: 4.1g; Fiber: 0.9g; Sugar: 3g

Turkey Meatballs Soup

Serves: 6 / Preparation time: 20 minutes / Cooking time:

25 minutes

For Meatballs

1 pound lean ground turkey 1 garlic clove, minced

1 organic egg, beaten ¼ cup Parmesan cheese,

grated

Salt and ground black pepper, as required

For Soup

1 tablespoon olive oil 1 small yellow onion,

chopped finely

1 garlic clove, minced 6 cups homemade chicken

broth

6 cups fresh kale, trimmed and chopped 2 organic eggs, beaten

lightly

¼ cup Parmesan cheese, grated Salt and ground black

pepper, as required

- For meatballs: in a bowl, add all the ingredients and mix until well

combined.

- Make small equal sized balls from the mixture.
- In a large soup pan, heat the oil over medium heat and sauté the

onion for about 5-6 minutes.

- Add the garlic and sauté for about 1 minute.
- Add the broth and bring to a boil.
- Carefully, place the balls in pan and bring to a boil.
- Reduce the heat to low and simmer for about 10 minutes.
- Stir in the kale and bring to a gentle simmer.
- Simmer for about 2-3 minutes.
- Slowly, add the beaten eggs, stirring continuously.
- Stir in the cheese until melted.
- Season with salt and black pepper and serve hot.
- Meal Prep Tip: Transfer the soup into a large bowl and set aside to

cool. Divide the mixture into 6 containers evenly. Cover the

containers and refrigerate for 1-2 days. Reheat in the microwave

before serving.

One Serving: Net Carbs: 6.5g; Calories: 297; Total Fat: 14.3g; Sat. Fat:

6.1g; Protein: 23.7g; Carbs: 9g; Fiber: 2.5g; Sugar: 1.4g

Shrimp with Zucchini

Serves: 4 / Preparation time: 20 minutes / Cooking time: 6 minutes

2 tablespoons olive oil 2 tablespoons unsalted

butter

1 pound medium shrimp, peeled and deveined

1 small yellow onion, minced 4 garlic cloves, minced

¼ teaspoon red pepper flakes, crushed Salt and ground black pepper,

as required

¼ cup homemade chicken broth 2 tablespoons fresh lemon

juice

1 teaspoon fresh lemon zest, grated ½ pound zucchini, spiralized

with Blade C

2 tablespoons Parmesan cheese, grated

- In a large skillet, heat oil and butter over medium-high heat and cook

shrimp, onion, garlic, red pepper flakes, salt and black pepper for

about 2 minutes, stirring occasionally.

- Stir in broth, lemon juice and lemon zest and bring to a gentle boil.
- Stir in zucchini noodles and cook for about 1-2 minutes.
- Serve hot with the topping of Parmesan.
- Meal Prep Tip: Transfer the shrimp mixture into a large bowl and set

aside to cool completely. Divide the mixture into 4 containers evenly.

Cover the containers and refrigerate for about 1-2 days. Reheat in

the microwave before serving. Sprinkle with the cheese just before

serving.

One Serving: Net Carbs: 3.3g; Calories: 274; Total Fat: 16.4g; Sat. Fat: 6g;

Protein: 28.8g; Carbs: 5.4g; Fiber: 1.2g; Sugar: 2g

Cheesy Pork Casserole

Serves: 8 / Preparation time: 20 minutes / Cooking time: 1¼ hours

For Pork

2 pounds ground pork 1 cup cheddar cheese,

shredded

1 tablespoon dried onion, minced 1 teaspoon dried garlic,

minced

1 teaspoon red chili powder 1 teaspoon garlic powder

1 teaspoon ground mustard Salt, to taste

1 organic egg 2 ounce sugar-free BBQ sauce

For Topping

2 ounces sugar-free BBQ sauce 5 cooked bacon slices,

chopped

½ cup cheddar cheese, shredded

- Preheat the oven to 400 degrees F. Greased a 9x13-inch casserole

dish.

- For pork mixture: in a bowl, add all the ingredients and mix until well combined.

• Place the mixture into the prepared casserole dish evenly and press

to smooth the surface.

• Coat the top of meatloaf with BBQ sauce evenly and sprinkle with

bacon, followed by the cheese.

• Bake for about 40 minutes.

• Remove the casserole from the oven and place onto a wire rack to

cool slightly.

• Cut into desired sized slices and serve warm.

• Meal Prep Tip: Remove the casserole from oven and set aside to cool

completely. Transfer the casserole slices onto a wire rack to cool

completely. With 1 piece of foil, wrap each slice and refrigerate for

about 1-2 days. Reheat in the microwave before serving.

One Serving: Net Carbs: 5.7g; Calories: 439; Total Fat: 23.9g; Sat. Fat:

10g; Protein: 46.6g; Carbs: 6g; Fiber: 0.3g; Sugar: 4g

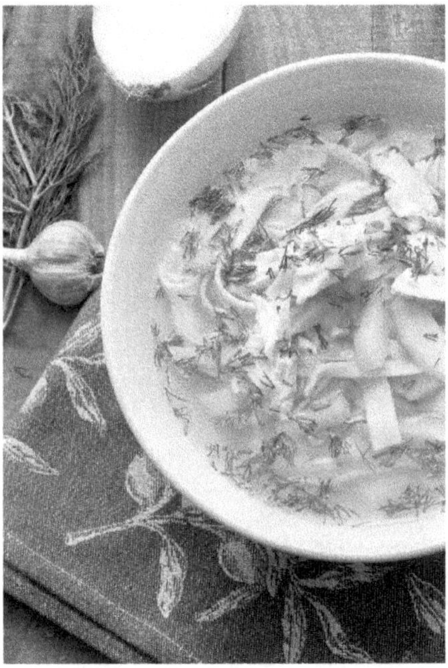

Chicken Soup

Serves: 4 / Preparation time: 20 minutes / Cooking time: 30 minutes

2 tablespoons butter 1 medium carrot, peeled and

chopped

½ cup yellow onion, chopped 2 celery stalks, chopped

1 garlic clove, minced 2 teaspoons xanthan gum

1 teaspoon dried parsley, crushed 1 teaspoon ground black

pepper

4 cups homemade chicken broth 12 ounces cauliflower,

chopped

2 cups cooked grass-fed chicken, chopped 2 cups heavy cream

¼ cup fresh parsley, chopped

- In a large soup pan, melt the butter over medium heat and sauté the

carrot, onion and celery for about 4-5 minutes.

- Add the garlic and sauté for about 1 minute.
- Meanwhile, in a bowl, mix together xanthan gum, parsley

and black

pepper.

- Stir in the parsley mixture, broth and cauliflower and bring to a boil.

- Reduce the heat to low and simmer, covered for about 20 minutes,

stirring occasionally.

- Stir in cooked chicken, cream, parsley and salt and simmer for about

3-4 minutes.

- Serve hot.

- Meal Prep Tip: Transfer the soup into a large bowl and set aside to

cool. Divide the mixture into 6 containers evenly. Cover the

containers and refrigerate for 1-2 days. Reheat in the microwave

before serving.

One Serving: Net Carbs: 4.6g; Calories: 280; Total Fat: 20.2g; Sat. Fat:

12.1g; Protein: 17.2g; Carbs: 7g; Fiber: 2.7g; Sugar: 2.4g

Bacon & Avocado Soup

Serves: 6 / Preparation time: 15 minutes / Cooking time: 5 minutes

4 cups homemade chicken broth 2 avocados, peeled, pitted

and chopped

1/3 cups fresh cilantro, chopped roughly ½ teaspoon garlic, chopped

roughly

1 teaspoon fresh lime juice ½ pound cooked bacon, chopped

Salt and ground black pepper, as required

- In a large pan, add the broth and bring to a boil.
- Reduce the heat to low.
- In a blender, add avocadoes, cilantro, garlic and lime juice and pulse

until chopped finely.

- Add 1 cup of the chicken broth and pulse until smooth.
- Transfer the avocado mixture into the pan of remaining simmering

broth and stir to combine.

- Stir in bacon, salt and pepper and remove from the heat.
- Serve immediately.
- Meal Prep Tip: Transfer the soup into a large bowl and set aside to

cool. Divide the soup into 6 airtight containers. Cover and refrigerate

for 1-2 days. Reheat in the microwave before serving.

One Serving: Net Carbs: 2.4g; Calories: 352; Total Fat: 28.9g; Sat. Fat:

7.9g; Protein: 16.6g; Carbs: 7g; Fiber: 4.6g; Sugar: 0.4g

Berries & Spinach Salad

Serves: 5 / Preparation time: 15 minutes

For Salad

8 ounces fresh baby spinach ¾ cup fresh strawberries,

hulled and sliced

¾ cup fresh blueberries ¼ cup feta cheese, crumbled

For Dressing

1/3 cup olive oil 2 tablespoons fresh lemon

juice

¼ teaspoon liquid stevia 1/8 teaspoon paprika

1/8 teaspoon garlic powder Salt, as required

- For salad: in a bowl, add the spinach, berries and almonds.

- For dressing: in another small bowl, add all the ingredients and beat

until well combined.

- Place the dressing over salad and gently, toss to coat well.

- Meal Prep Tip: In the bottom of 4 large mason jars, divide the

dressing. Place the salad ingredients in this order:

strawberries,

followed by blueberries, spinach and almonds. Cover each jar with

the lid tightly and refrigerate for about 1 day. Shake the jars well just

before serving.

One Serving: Net Carbs: 4.4g; Calories: 167; Total Fat: 15.4g; Sat. Fat:

3.1g; Protein: 2.8g; Carbs: 7g; Fiber: 2.6g; Sugar: 3.9g

Chicken Burgers

Serves: 4 / Preparation time: 15 minutes / Cooking time: 10 minutes

1¼ pounds grass-fed ground chicken 1 organic egg

½ yellow onion, grated Salt and ground black pepper,

as required

1 teaspoon dried thyme 3 tablespoons butter

- n a bowl, add all the ingredients and mix until well combined.

- Make 8 small equal sized patties from the mixture.

- In a large frying pan, melt butter over medium heat and cook the

patties for about 4-5 minutes per side or until done completely.

- Serve hot.

- Meal Prep Tip: Remove the patties from heat and set aside to cool

completely. Store in an airtight container, by placing parchment

papers between the burgers to avoid the sticking. These burgers can

be stored in the freezer for up to 3 weeks. Before serving, thaw the

burgers and then reheat in microwave.

One Serving: Net Carbs: 1.1g; Calories: 368; Total Fat: 20.7g; Sat. Fat:

8.7g; Protein: 42.7g; Carbs: 1.5g; Fiber: 0.4g; Sugar: 0.7g

Turkey Salad

Serves: 5 / Preparation time: 15 minutes / Cooking time: 13 minutes

1 tablespoon olive oil 1 pound ground turkey

Salt and ground black pepper, as required ¼ cup water

1 English cucumber, chopped 4 cups green cabbage,

shredded

½ cup fresh mint leaves, chopped 2 tablespoons fresh lime

juice

¼ cup walnuts, chopped

- In a large skillet, heat oil over medium-high heat and cook turkey for

about 6-8 minutes.

- Stir in water and cook for about 4-5 minutes or until almost all the

liquid is evaporated.

- Transfer turkey into a bowl and set aside to cool.
- In a large bowl, mix together remaining ingredients.
- Add the turkey and stir to combine.
- Meal Prep Tip: In 5 containers, divide turkey and salad evenly and

refrigerate for about 1 day.

One Serving: Net Carbs: 4.1g; Calories: 267; Total Fat: 16.7g; Sat. Fat:

2.3g; Protein: 27.7g; Carbs: 6.9g; Fiber: 2.8g; Sugar: 2.9g

Beef Stew

Serves: 8 / Preparation time: 15 minutes / Cooking time: 2 hours 10

minutes

2 pounds grass-fed beef stew meat, trimmed and cubed into 1-inch size

1 1/3 cups homemade hot chicken broth 2 yellow onions, chopped

2 bay leaves 1 teaspoon Greek seasoning

Ground black pepper, as required 3 celery stalks, chopped

1 (8-ounce) package shredded cabbage 1 (8-ounce) can sugar-free

tomato sauce

1 (8-ounce) can sugar-free whole plum tomatoes, chopped roughly with

liquid

Salt, to taste

- Heat a large nonstick pan over medium-high heat and cook the beef

for about 4-5 minutes or until browned.

- Drain excess grease from the pan.
- Stir in the broth, onion, bay leaves, Greek seasoning and black

pepper and bring to a boil.

- Reduce the heat to low and simmer, covered for about 1¼ hours.
- Stir in celery and cabbage and simmer, covered for about 30 minutes.
- Stir in the tomato sauce and chopped plum tomatoes and simmer,

uncovered for about 15-20 minutes.

- Stir in the salt and remove from heat.
- Discard bay leaves and serve hot.
- Meal Prep Tip: Transfer the stew into a large bowl and set aside to

cool. Divide the stew into 8 containers evenly. Cover the containers

and refrigerate for 1-2 days. Reheat in the microwave before serving.

One Serving: Net Carbs: 2.4g; Calories: 250; Total Fat: 7.5; Sat. Fat: 2.8g;

Protein: 36.7g; Carbs: 7g; Fiber: 2.1g; Sugar: 4.6g

Grouper Curry

Serves: 4 / Preparation time: 15 minutes / Cooking time: 15 minutes

1½ pounds skinless grouper fillets, cubed into 2-inch size

1 tablespoon coconut oil 1 small yellow onion,

chopped

2 garlic cloves, minced 1 teaspoon fresh ginger,

minced

1 large tomato, peeled and chopped 1½ tablespoons red curry

paste

¼ cup water 1¼ cups unsweetened

coconut milk

Salt, to taste 2 tablespoons fresh basil

leaves, chopped

- In a large skillet, heat the oil over medium heat and sauté the onion,

garlic and ginger for about 5 minutes.

- Add the tomatoes and cook for about 2-3 minutes, crushing with the

back of spoon.

- Add the curry paste and sauté for about 2 minutes.
- Add the water and coconut milk and bring to a gentle boil.
- Stir in the grouper and cook for about 4-5 minutes.
- Stir in salt and basil leaves and serve hot.
- Meal Prep Tip: Transfer the curry into a large bowl and set aside to

cool. Divide the curry into 4 containers evenly. Cover the containers

and refrigerate for 1-2 days. Reheat in the microwave before serving.

One Serving: Net Carbs: 4.6g; Calories: 286; Total Fat: 8.7g; Sat. Fat:

5.3g; Protein: 43g; Carbs: 6g; Fiber: 1.4g; Sugar: 2g

Chicken with Spinach

Serves: 4 / Preparation time: 15 minutes / Cooking time: 13 minutes

2 tablespoons butter, divided 1 pound grass-fed chicken

tenders

Salt and ground black pepper, as required 2 garlic cloves, minced

1 jalapeño pepper, chopped 10 ounces frozen spinach,

thawed

¼ cup Parmesan cheese, shredded ¼ cup heavy cream

• In a large skillet, melt 1 tablespoon of the butter over medium-high

heat and cook the chicken with salt and black pepper for about 2-3

minutes per side.

• Transfer the chicken into a bowl.

• In the same skillet, melt remaining butter over medium-low heat and sauté the garlic for about 1 minute.

- Add the spinach and cook for about 1 minute.
- Add the cheese, cream, salt and black pepper and stir to combine.
- Spread the spinach mixture in the bottom of skillet evenly.
- Place chicken over spinach in a single layer.
- Immediately, reduce the heat to low and simmer, covered for about 5

minutes.

- Serve hot.
- Meal Prep Tip: Transfer the chicken mixture into a large bowl and set

aside to cool completely. Divide the mixture into 4 containers evenly.

Cover the containers and refrigerate for up to 2 days. Reheat in the

microwave before serving.

One Serving: Net Carbs: 2g; Calories: 333; Total Fat: 18.6g; Sat. Fat: 8.6g;

Protein: 37.1g; Carbs: 3.7g; Fiber: 1.7g; Sugar: 0.5g

Broccoli Soup

Serves: 5 / Preparation time: 15 minutes / Cooking time: 15 minutes

4 cups homemade chicken broth 20 ounces small broccoli

florets

12 ounces cheddar cheese, cubed Salt and ground black

pepper, as required

1 cup heavy cream

- In a large soup pan, add the broth and broccoli over medium-high

heat and bring to a boil.

- Reduce the heat to low and simmer, covered for about 5-7 minutes.
- Stir in the cheese and simmer for about 2-3 minutes, stirring

continuously.

- Stir in the salt, black pepper and cream and simmer for about 2

minutes.

- Serve hot.
- Meal Prep Tip: Transfer the soup into a large bowl and

set aside to

cool. Divide the soup into 4 airtight containers. Cover and refrigerate

for 1-2 days. Reheat in the microwave before serving.

One Serving: Net Carbs: 5g; Calories: 403; Total Fat: 32.2g; Sat. Fat: 20g;

Protein: 21.2g; Carbs: 8g; Fiber: 3g; Sugar: 2.9g

Salmon Burgers

Serves: 8 / Preparation time: 15 minutes / Cooking time: 20 minutes

1 organic egg 3 tablespoons sugar-free

ranch dressing

1 (14-ounce) can pink salmon, drained and bones removed

2 ounces smoked salmon, chopped roughly 1/3 cup almond flour

2 tablespoons fresh parsley, chopped 1 teaspoon Cajun seasoning

2 tablespoons avocado oil

- In a large bowl, add the egg and ranch dressing and beat until well

combined.

- Add the remaining ingredients and gently, mix until well combined.
- Make 8 equal sized patties from the mixture.
- In a nonstick skillet, heat oil over medium heat and cook the patties in

2 batches for about 3-5 minutes per side or until golden brown.

- Serve hot.
- Meal Prep Tip: Remove the patties from heat and set aside to cool

completely. Store in an airtight container, by placing parchment papers between the burgers to avoid the sticking. These burgers can

be stored in the freezer for up to 3 weeks. Before serving, thaw the

burgers and then reheat in microwave.

One Serving: Net Carbs: 0.6g; Calories: 106; Total Fat: 6.2g; Sat. Fat:

0.8g; Protein: 12g; Carbs: 1.3g; Fiber: 0.7g; Sugar: 0.2g

Chicken Meatballs with Guacamole

Serves: 6 / Preparation time: 20 minutes / Cooking time: 18 minutes

For Meatballs:

1 pound grass-fed lean ground chicken 2 ounces cheddar cheese,

grated

2 tablespoons almond flour 2 tablespoons golden flax

meal

½ of medium red bell pepper, seeded and chopped

2 medium scallions, chopped 2 tablespoons fresh cilantro,

chopped

1 teaspoon fresh lime zest, grated finely 1 tablespoon fresh lime juice

½ teaspoon garlic powder ½ teaspoon red pepper

flakes, crushed

For Guacamole

1 large avocado, peeled, pitted and chopped

1 tablespoon fresh lime juice ¼ teaspoon garlic powder

Salt and ground black pepper, as required

- Preheat the oven to 350 degrees F. Grease a large baking sheet.
- For meatballs: in a bowl, add all the ingredients and mix until well

combined.

- Make equal sized meatballs from chicken mixture.
- Arrange balls onto prepared baking sheet and bake for about 15-18

minutes.

- Meanwhile, for guacamole: in a bowl, add all ingredients and with a

fork, mash until well combined.

- Serve meatballs alongside guacamole.

- Meal Prep Tip: Transfer the meatballs onto a large platter and set

aside to cool completely. Then, arrange the meatballs onto a

parchment paper lined freezer-safe platter and freeze or about 1-2

hours. Now, divide the meatballs into reseal able plastic bags. Seal

the bags and freeze for 1-2 weeks. In an airtight container, place the

guacamole and with a spoon remove any air pockets. Then, flatten

the top surface completely. Gently place about ½- inch of water on

top to cover the guacamole surface. Cover tightly and refrigerate up

to 2 days. Thaw the meatballs before serving. Preheat the oven to

350 degrees F. arrange the meatballs onto a greased baking dish ina single layer and bake until heated through. Just before serving,

carefully pour off the water from the container of the guacamole.

Then, gently stir the guacamole and serve alongside the heated

meatballs.

One Serving: Net Carbs: 2.3g; Calories: 282; Total Fat: 17.3g; Sat. Fat: 5g;

Protein: 26.1g; Carbs: 5.8g; Fiber: 3.5g; Sugar: 1g

Chicken Chili

Serves: 12 / Preparation time: 15 minutes / Cooking time: 1¾ hours

2 tablespoons olive oil 1 large yellow onion,

chopped

2 medium green bell peppers, seeded and chopped

4 garlic cloves, minced 1 jalapeño pepper, chopped

1 teaspoon dried basil 1 teaspoon dried thyme

2 tablespoons red chili powder 1 tablespoon ground cumin

2½ pounds grass-fed ground chicken 8 ounces sugar-free tomato

paste

2 cups homemade chicken broth 2 cups water

Salt and ground black pepper, as required

• In a large pan, heat the oil over medium heat and sauté the onion and

bell pepper for about 5-7 minutes.

• Add the garlic, jalapeño pepper, herbs, spices and black pepper and

sauté for about 1 minute.

• Add the chicken and cook for about 4-5 minutes.

• Stir in the tomato paste and cook for about 2 minutes.

• Add the broth and water and bring to a boil.

• Reduce the heat to low and simmer, covered for about 1-1½ hours or

until desired doneness.

• Stir in the salt and black pepper and serve hot.

• Meal Prep Tip: Transfer the chili into a large bowl and set aside to cool. Divide the chili into 12 containers evenly. Cover the containers

and refrigerate for 6-7 days. Reheat in the microwave before serving.

One Serving: Net Carbs: 5.6g; Calories: 240; Total Fat: 9.9g; Sat. Fat:

2.

Beef & Veggie Wraps

Serves: 6 / Preparation time: 15 minutes / Cooking time: 20 minutes

2 tablespoons unsalted butter 1 pound lean ground beef

1 yellow onion, chopped 2 garlic cloves, minced

1 bell pepper, seeded and chopped 1 cup carrot, peeled and

chopped

½ cup yellow squash, chopped ½ cup zucchini, chopped

2 tablespoons low-sodium soy sauce ½ teaspoon curry powder

Ground black pepper, as required 12 lettuce leaves

1½ cups Parmesan cheese, shredded

- In a large skillet, melt the butter over medium heat and cook the beef

for about 8-10 minutes, breaking the lumps.

- Stir in the vegetables and cook for about 4-5 minutes.
- Stir in the soy sauce, curry powder and black pepper and cook for

about 4-5 minutes.

- Remove from the heat and set aside to cool slightly.
- Arrange lettuce leaves onto serving plates and top each with beef

mixture evenly.

- Sprinkle with cheese and serve.
- Meal Prep Tip: Remove the turkey mixture from heat and set aside to

cool completely. In 10 containers, divide the beef mixture evenly and

refrigerate for about 2 days. Reheat slightly in microwave before

serving. Divide the turkey mixture over the lettuce leaves evenly. Top

with the cheese and serve.

One Serving: Net Carbs: 5.5g; Calories: 287; Total Fat: 14.2g; Sat. Fat:

7.7g; Protein: 31.8g; Carbs: 7g; Fiber: 1.5g; Sugar: 3.5g

Lobster Salad

Serves: 16 / Preparation time: 20 minutes

5 pounds cooked lobster meat, shredded 7 celery stalks, chopped

3 yellow bell peppers, seeded and chopped 1 large yellow onion,

chopped

2 cups mayonnaise Ground black pepper, as

required

- In a large bowl, add all ingredients and mix until well combined.

- Refrigerate to chill before serving.

- Meal Prep Tip: In 16 containers, divide salad and refrigerate for about

1 day.

One Serving: Net Carbs: 1.7g; Calories: 219; Total Fat: 21.3g; Sat. Fat:

3.3g; Protein: 27.3g; Carbs: 2.4g; Fiber: 0.7g; Sugar: 1.6g

Savory Zucchini Cake

Serves: 8 / Preparation time: 15 minutes / Cooking time: 52 minutes

2 tablespoons olive oil 1 large zucchini, grated

6 large organic eggs (whites and yolks separated)

2 scallions, chopped 2 tablespoons fresh

mint leaves, chopped

½ cup Parmesan cheese, grated ½ cup feta cheese, crumbled

½ cup coconut flour ½ teaspoon organic baking

powder

1 teaspoon garlic powder Salt and ground black

pepper, as required

- Preheat the oven to 400 degrees F. Line the bottom of a

greased

spring form pan with parchment paper.

• In a frying pan, heat oil over medium heat and cook the zucchini for

about 10-12 minutes, stirring occasionally.

• Remove from the heat and set aside to cool slightly.

• Meanwhile, in a bowl, add the egg whites and beat until stiff peaks

form.

• In another bowl, add the zucchini, egg yolks and remaining

ingredients and mix until well combined.

• Gently fold in the whipped egg whites.

• Place the mixture into the prepared pan evenly.

• Bake for about 40 minutes.

• Remove from the oven and set aside to cool for about 10 minutes

before serving.

• Cut into 8 equal sized wedges and serve.

• Meal Prep Tip: In a reseal able plastic bag, place the

cooled cake

slices and seal the bag. Refrigerate for about 2-4 days. Reheat in the

microwave on High for about 1 minute before serving.

One Serving: Net Carbs: 2.6g; Calories: 173; Total Fat: 13g; Sat. Fat: 5.6g;

Protein: 12.1g; Carbs: 3.4g; Fiber: 0.8g; Sugar: 1.3g

Green Beans with Mushrooms

Serves: 4 / Preparation time: 15 minutes / Cooking time: 16 minutes

2 tablespoons butter 2 tablespoons onion, minced

½ teaspoon garlic, minced 1 teaspoon fresh rosemary,

minced

1 (8-ounce) package white mushrooms, sliced

2 cooked bacon slices, crumbled Pinch of salt

1 cup frozen green beans

- In a large skillet, melt butter over medium heat and sauté the onion

and garlic for about 1 minute.

- Add the mushrooms and cook for about 5 minutes.
- Stir in the bacon and salt and cook for about 5 minutes.
- Stir in the green beans and cook for about 5 minutes or until desired

doneness.

- Serve hot.

• Meal Prep Tip: Transfer the green beans and tomatoes into a large

bowl and set aside to cool completely. Divide the mixture into 4

containers evenly. Cover the containers and refrigerate for about 2

days. Reheat in the microwave before serving.

One Serving: Net Carbs: 2.4g; Calories: 153; Total Fat: 12g; Sat. Fat: 5.7g;

Protein: 7.8g; Carbs: 4g; Fiber: 1.6g; Sugar: 1.6g

Steak Salad

Serves: 5 / Preparation time: 20 minutes / Cooking time: 12 minutes

For Salad

1 tablespoon low-sodium soy sauce 1 teaspoon Montreal steak

seasoning

1 (12-ounce) grass-fed rib-eye steak 2 medium carrots, peeled and

grated

2 English cucumbers, cubed 2 large tomatoes,

chopped

¼ cup red onion, chopped 3 cups romaine lettuce

leaves, torn

For Dressing

3 tablespoons olive oil 3 tablespoons fresh lemon

juice

1 tablespoons Erythritol ¼ teaspoon garlic powder

1/8 teaspoon red pepper flakes, crushed

- For steak: in a large bowl, mix together the soy sauce and steak

seasoning.

- Add the steak and coat with seasoning mixture evenly.

- Cover and refrigerate to marinate for at least 1 hour.

- Preheat the grill to medium-high heat. Grease the grill grate.
- Grill the steak for about 6 minutes per side.
- Remove from grill and place the steak onto a cutting board.
- Set aside for about 10 minutes before slicing.
- With a sharp knife, cut the beef steak diagonally into slices across

grain.

- Set aside to cool completely.
- In a large bowl, mix together remaining salad ingredients.
- In another bowl, add all dressing ingredients and beat until well

combined.

- Place the dressing over salad and gently toss to coat well.
- In a small, jar, place the reserved marinade. In 4 containers, divide

salad and steak slices. Refrigerate the containers and jar of dressing

for about 1 day. Just before serving, place the dressing over the salad and toss to coat well.

One Serving: Net Carbs: 7g; Calories: 312; Total Fat: 23.9g; Sat. Fat: 7.4g;

Protein: 14.2g; Carbs: 10g; Fiber: 3g; Sugar: 6g

Pork Stew

Serves: 8 / Preparation time: 15 minutes / Cooking time: 1 hour 35 minutes

1 (4-ounce) can whole hatch green chilies with liquid

½ cup yellow onion, chopped 2 garlic cloves, chopped

3 tablespoons olive oil 2 pounds pork loin,

trimmed and cubed

2 teaspoons ground cumin 1 teaspoon ground

coriander

1 teaspoon red chili powder Salt and ground black

pepper, as required

2½ cups homemade chicken broth

- In a food processor, add the green chilies with juice, onion and garlic

and pulse until a thick chunky paste is formed.

- In a large pan, heat the oil over medium heat and cook the pork for

about 4-5 minutes or until browned completely.

- Add the spices and cook for about 1 minute.
- Add the chilies paste and broth and bring to a boil.
- Reduce the heat to low and simmer, covered for about 1-1½ hours.
- Serve hot.
- Meal Prep Tip: Transfer the stew into a large bowl and

set aside to

cool. Divide the stew into 8 containers evenly. Cover the containers

and refrigerate for 1-2 days. Reheat in the microwave before serving.

One Serving: Net Carbs: 1.7; Calories: 341; Total Fat: 21.7g; Sat. Fat:

6.8g; Protein: 32.9g; Carbs: 2.3g; Fiber: 0.6g; Sugar: 0.6g

Turkey Chili

Serves: 5 / Preparation time: 15 minutes / Cooking time: 25 minutes

2 tablespoons coconut oil ½ yellow onion, chopped

finely

2 garlic cloves, minced 1 pound ground turkey

2 cups cauliflower, processed into rice consistency

2 cups heavy cream 1 tablespoon mustard

1 tablespoon red chili powder 1 teaspoon dried thyme

Salt and ground black pepper, as required

- In a large pan, melt the coconut oil over medium heat and sauté the

onion and garlic for about 2-3 minutes.

- Add the turkey and cook for about 8-10 minutes.
- Stir in remaining all ingredients and bring to a boil.
- Reduce the heat to low and simmer, covered for about 10-12

minutes.

- Serve hot.
- Meal Prep Tip: Transfer the chili into a large bowl and set aside to

cool. Divide the chili into 5 containers evenly. Cover the containers

and refrigerate for 6-7 days. Reheat in the microwave

before serving.

One Serving: Net Carbs: 4g; Calories: 421; Total Fat: 34.1g; Sat. Fat:

17.5g; Protein: 27.6g; Carbs: 6.2g; Fiber: 2.2g; Sugar: 1.8g

Steak in Mushroom Sauce

Serves: 8 / Preparation time: 15 minutes / Cooking time: 10 minutes

1 (2-pound) grass-fed flat iron steak Salt and ground black

pepper, as required

2 tablespoons olive oil 1 large yellow onion, sliced

thinly

½ cup Italian dressing 2 Portobello mushrooms,

sliced

3 large red bell peppers, seeded and sliced thinly

1/3 cup homemade chicken broth ½ cup blue cheese,

crumbled

Preheat the grill to medium-high heat. Grease the grill grate.

- Sprinkle the steak with salt and black pepper generously.
- Grill the steak for about 5 minutes per side.
- Transfer the steak onto a cutting board and set aside for about 10

minutes before slicing.

- With a sharp knife, cut the steak into desired size slices diagonally

across grain.

- Meanwhile, in a skillet, heat the oil over medium-high heat and sauté

the onion for about 4 minutes.

- Add Italian dressing and bring to a boil.
- Add the mushrooms and bell pepper and stir to combine.
- Reduce the heat to medium and cook for about 5 minutes, stirring

occasionally.

- With a slotted spoon, transfer the vegetables into a bowl.
- Add the broth in skillet and immediately increase the heat to medium high.
- Cook for about 5 minutes or until desired thickness of sauce, stirring

frequently.

- Divide vegetable mixture onto serving plates and top with steak

slices.

- Sprinkle with cheese and serve.
- Meal Prep Tip: Transfer the steak and vegetables into a large bowl

and set aside to cool completely. Divide the mixture into 6 containers

evenly. Cover the containers and refrigerate for up to 3-4 days.

Reheat in the microwave before serving.

One Serving: Net Carbs: 5.2g; Calories: 364; Total Fat: 19.4g; Sat. Fat:

7.3g; Protein: 39.1g; Carbs: 7g; Fiber: 1.8g; Sugar: 4g

Stuffed Leg of Lamb

Serves: 14 / Preparation time: 20 minutes / Cooking time: 1¾ hours

1/3 cup fresh parsley, minced finely 8 garlic cloves, minced

and divided

3 tablespoons olive oil, divided Salt and ground black

pepper, as required

1 (4-pound) gras `s-fed boneless leg of lamb, butterflied and trimmed

1/3 cup yellow onion, minced 4 cups fresh kale,

trimmed and chopped

½ cup Kalamata olives, pitted and chopped ½ cup feta cheese,

crumbled

1 teaspoon fresh lemon zest, grated finely

- In a large baking dish, mix together the parsley, 4 garlic cloves, 2

tablespoons of oil, salt and black pepper.

- Add the leg of lamb and coat with parsley mixture generously.
- Set aside in the room temperature.
- Preheat the oven to 450 degrees F. Grease a shallow roasting pan.
- In a large skillet, heat the remaining oil over medium heat.
- Add the onion and remaining garlic and sauté for about 3-5 minutes.
- Add the kale and cook for about 8-10 minutes.
- Remove from the heat and set aside to cool for at least 10 minutes.
- Stir in the remaining ingredients.

- Place the leg of lamb onto a smooth surface, cut-side up.
- Place the kale mixture in the center, leaving 1-inch border from both

sides.

- Roll the short side to seal the stuffing.
- With a kitchen string tightly, tie the roll at many places.
- Arrange the rolled leg of lamb into the prepared roasting pan, seam side down.
- Roast for about 15 minutes.
- Now, reduce the temperature of oven to 350 degrees F.
- Roast for about 1-1¼ hours.
- Remove the leg of lamb from oven and set aside for about 10-20

minutes before slicing.

- With a sharp knife, cut the roll into desired size slices and serve.
- Meal Prep Tip: Transfer the lamb slices onto a wire rack to cool

completely. With foil pieces, wrap the lamb slices and refrigerate for

about 1-2 days. Reheat in the microwave before

serving.One Serving: Net Carbs: 2.9g; Calories: 300; Total Fat: 14.2g; Sat. Fat:

4.7g; Protein: 37.9g; Carbs: 3.5g; Fiber: 0.6g; Sugar: 0.4g

Cabbage Bake

Serves: 3 / Preparation time: 15 minutes / Cooking time: 10 minutes

½ head green cabbage 2 scallions, chopped

4 tablespoons unsalted butter 2 ounces cream cheese,

softened

¼ cup Parmesan cheese, grated ¼ cup cream

½ teaspoon Dijon mustard 2 tablespoons fresh parsley,

chopped

Salt and ground black pepper, as required

• Preheat the oven to 350 degrees F.

• Cut cabbage head in half, lengthwise. Then cut into 4 equal sized

wedges.

• In a pan of boiling water, add cabbage wedges and simmer, covered

for about 5 minutes.

• Drain well and arrange cabbage wedges in a small baking dish.

• In a small pan, melt butter and sauté onions for about 5 minutes.

• Add the remaining ingredients and stir to combine.

• Remove from the heat and immediately, place the cheese mixture

over cabbage wedges evenly.

• Bake for about 20 minutes.

• Remove from the oven and set aside to cool for about 5 minutes

before serving.

- Cut into 3 equal sized portions and serve.
- Meal Prep Tip: Remove the baking dish from oven and set aside to

cool completely. Divide the mixture into 3 containers evenly. Cover

the containers and refrigerate for about 2 days. Reheat in the

microwave before serving.

One Serving: Net Carbs: 4.5g; Calories: 273; Total Fat: 24.8g; Sat. Fat:

15.4g; Protein: 6.2g; Carbs: 8g; Fiber: 3.5g; Sugar: 4.5g

Cheese Stuffed Turkey Burgers

Serves: 2 / Preparation time: 15 minutes / Cooking time: 6 minutes

8 ounces ground turkey Salt and ground black

pepper, as required

1 ounce mozzarella cheese, cubed 1 tablespoon butter

- In a bowl, add all the turkey, salt and black pepper and mix until well

combined.

- Make 2 equal sized patties from the mixture.

- Place mozzarella cubes inside each patty and cover with the beef.

- In a frying pan, melt butter over medium heat and cook patties for

about 2-3 minutes per side.

- Serve hot.

- Meal Prep Tip: Remove the patties from heat and set aside to cool completely. Store in an airtight container, by placing parchment

papers between the burgers to avoid the sticking. These burgers can

be stored iin the refrigerator for about 1 day. Before serving, reheat in

microwave.

One Serving: Net Carbs: 0.5g; Calories: 312; Total Fat: 20.7g; Sat. Fat:

7.2g; Protein: 35.1g; Carbs: 0.5g; Fiber: 0g; Sugar: 0gShrimp Salad

Serves: 6 / Preparation time: 20 minutes / Cooking time: 4 minutes

For Dressing

2 tablespoons butter 1 garlic clove, crushed

1 tablespoon fresh cilantro, chopped 1 tablespoon yacon

syrup

1 tablespoon fresh lime juice 2 teaspoons balsamic vinegar

½ teaspoon cayenne pepper ¼ teaspoon

salt

1 tablespoon water 1/3 cup olive oil

For Salad:

1 pound shrimp, peeled and deveined Salt and ground black

pepper, as required

1 teaspoon olive oil 1 cup carrots, peeled and

julienned

½ cup red cabbage, shredded ½ cup purple cabbage,

shredded

1 cup cucumber, julienned 2 cups fresh baby

arugula

2 cups lettuce, torn ¼ cup fresh basil,

chopped

¼ cup fresh cilantro, chopped

- For dressing: in a bowl, add all the ingredients except the oil and beat

until well combined.

- Slowly, add the oil, beating continuously until smooth.

- For salad: in a bowl, add the shrimp, salt, black pepper and oil and

toss to coat well.

- Heat a skillet over medium-high heat and cook the shrimp for about 2

minutes per side.

- Remove from the heat and set aside to cool.

- In a large bowl, add the shrimp and remaining ingredients and mix.

- Place the dressing over salad and gently, toss to coat well.

- Serve immediately.

- Meal Prep Tip: Divide dressing in 6 large mason jars evenly. Place

the remaining ingredients in in this order: carrots, cabbage,cucumber, arugula, basil, cilantro, shrimp and lettuce. Cover each jar

with the lid tightly and refrigerate for about 1 day. Shake the jars well

just before serving.

One Serving: Net Carbs: 5g; Calories: 242; Total Fat: 16.5g; Sat. Fat: 4.4g;

Protein: 18g; Carbs: 7g; Fiber: 2g; Sugar: 3.1g

Bacon & Tomato Salad

Serves: 3 / Preparation time: 15 minutes

For Dressing

½ cup mayonnaise 3 teaspoons fresh lemon juice

8-10 drops liquid stevia Ground black pepper, as

required

For Salad

4 cups romaine lettuce, chopped 2 tomatoes, chopped

½ pound cooked bacon, chopped

- For dressing: in a bowl, add all the ingredients and mix until well

combined.

- For salad: in a larger bowl, add all the ingredients admix well.
- Place the dressing over the salad and gently toss to coat well.
- Serve immediately.
- Meal Prep Tip: In a small, jar, place the dressing. In 4

containers,

divide the salad ingredients. Refrigerate the salad and dressing for

about 1-2 days. Just before serving, place the dressing over salad

and toss to coat well.

One Serving: Net Carbs: 5g; Calories: 675; Total Fat: 58.6g; Sat. Fat:

14.5g; Protein: 29.1g; Carbs: 6.1g; Fiber: 1.5g; Sugar: 3zg

Tuna Burgers

Serves: 4 / Preparation time: 15 minutes / Cooking time: 6 minutes

1 (15-ounce) can water packed tuna, drained

½ celery stalk, chopped 2 tablespoons fresh parsley,

copped

1 teaspoon fresh dill, chopped 2 tablespoons walnuts,

chopped

2 tablespoons mayonnaise 1 organic egg, beaten

1 tablespoon butter ¼ cup cheddar cheese, shredded

- In a bowl, add all the ingredients except butter and cheese and mix

until well combined.

- Make 2 equal sized patties from the mixture.

- In a frying pan, melt butter over medium heat and cook the patties for

about 2-3 minutes.

- Carefully, flip the side and top each patty with cheese

evenly.

- Cook for about 2-3 minutes.

- Serve hot.

- Meal Prep Tip: Remove the patties from heat and set aside to cool

completely. Store in an airtight container, by placing parchment

papers between the burgers to avoid the sticking. These burgers can

be stored in the freezer for up to 3 weeks. Before serving, thaw the

burgers and then reheat in microwave.

One Serving: Net Carbs: 2.2g; Calories: 322; Total Fat: 19.7g; Sat. Fat:

5.9g; Protein: 32.5g; Carbs: 2.6g; Fiber: 0.4g; Sugar: 0.7g

Chicken Stew

Serves: 6 / Preparation time: 20 minutes / Cooking time: 35 minutes

3 tablespoons unsalted butter ½ cup yellow onion, chopped

¾ cup bell pepper, seeded and chopped 30 ounces homemade

chicken broth

1 bay leaf 2/3 cup fluid whipping cream

17 ounces asparagus, trimmed and cut into 2-inch pieces

8 ounces fresh mushrooms, sliced

1 cup fresh green beans, cut into 2-inch pieces

40 ounces cooked grass-fed boneless chicken, chopped

Salt and ground black pepper, as required 2 tablespoons fresh thyme,

minced

- In a large pan, melt the butter over medium heat and sauté the onion and bell pepper for about 4-5 minutes.

- Add the broth and bay leaf and bring to a boil.
- Cook for about 10 minutes.
- Meanwhile, in a small pan, add cream over medium heat and cook for

about 5-7 minutes, stirring occasionally.

- Add the asparagus, mushrooms and green beans into the pan of

broth mixture and cook for about 7 minutes.

- Add the cooked chicken and stir to combine.
- Reduce the heat to low and simmer for about 3 minutes.
- Stir in the salt, black pepper, thyme and cream and immediately,

remove from the heat.

- Serve hot.
- Meal Prep Tip: Transfer the stew into a large bowl and set aside to

cool. Divide the stew into 6 containers evenly. Cover the containers

and refrigerate for 1-2 days. Reheat in the microwave before serving.

One Serving: Net Carbs: 5.6g; Calories: 513; Total Fat: 25g; Sat. Fat:

10.4g; Protein: 61.5g; Carbs: 9g; Fiber: 3.4g; Sugar: 4g

Beef Curry

Serves: 6 / Preparation time: 15 minutes / Cooking time: 3 hours 25

minutes

2½ pounds grass-fed beef chuck roast, cubed into 1-inch size

2 tablespoons butter 3 tablespoons red curry

paste

2½ cups unsweetened coconut milk ½ cup homemade chicken

broth

Salt and ground black pepper, as required ¼ cup fresh cilantro,

chopped

- In a large pan, melt the butter over low heat and sauté the curry paste

for about 4-5 minutes.

- Stir in the coconut milk and broth and bring to a simmer.

- Simmer for about 4-5 minutes.

- Stir in the beef and bring to a boil over medium heat.

- Reduce the heat to low and simmer, covered for about 2½ hours,

stirring occasionally

- Remove from heat and with a slotted spoon, transfer the beef into a

bowl.

- Set the pan aside for about 10 minutes.

- With a slotted spoon, remove the fats from top of the curry.

- Return the pan over medium heat.

- Stir in the meat and bring to a gentle simmer.

- Reduce the heat to low and simmer, uncovered for about 30 minutes

or until desired thickness.

- Stir in the salt and remove from the heat.

- Serve hot with the garnishing of cilantro.

- Meal Prep Tip: Transfer the curry into a large bowl and set aside to cool. Divide the curry into 6 containers evenly. Cover the containers

and refrigerate for 1-2 days. Reheat in the microwave before serving.

One Serving: Net Carbs: 2g; Calories: 772; Total Fat: 60.5g; Sat. Fat:

25.8g; Protein: 49.9g; Carbs: 2.4g; Fiber: 0.4g; Sugar: 0.1g

Lamb Curry

Serves: 4 / Preparation time: 20 minutes / Cooking time: 1 hour 50 minutes

1 pound grass-fed boneless lamb, trimmed and cubed

Salt and ground black pepper, as required 2 teaspoons coconut oil

1 celery stalk, chopped 1 medium yellow onion,

chopped

1 Serrano pepper, chopped 1 teaspoon butter

2 garlic cloves, minced 1 teaspoon ground

cumin

1 teaspoon ground coriander ¼ teaspoon ground

turmeric

2 tablespoons sugar-free tomato paste 1 cup unsweetened

coconut milk

½ cup water 1 medium carrot, peeled

and chopped

1 teaspoon fresh lemon juice 2 tablespoons fresh

cilantro, chopped

• Season the lamb pieces with the salt and black pepper evenly.

• In a large pan, melt the coconut oil over high heat and sear lamb for

about 4-5 minutes.

• Add the onion, celery and Serrano and cook for about 1 minute.

• Reduce the heat to medium.

• Stir in the butter, garlic and spices and cook for about 1 minute.

• Stir in the tomato paste, coconut milk and water and

bring to a boil.

- Reduce the heat to low and simmer, covered for about 1 hour, stirring

occasionally.

- Stir in the carrot and simmer, covered for about 40 minutes.

- Stir in the lemon juice and salt and remove from heat.

- Serve hot with the garnishing of cilantro.

- Meal Prep Tip: Transfer the curry into a large bowl and set aside to

cool. Divide the curry into 4 containers evenly. Cover the containers

and refrigerate for 1-2 days. Reheat in the microwave before serving.

One Serving: Net Carbs: 4.2g; Calories: 290; Total Fat: 12.8g; Sat. Fat:

6.6g; Protein: 32.9g; Carbs: 6g; Fiber: 1.8g; Sugar: 3g

Steak with Blueberry Sauce

Serves: 4 / Preparation time: 15 minutes / Cooking time: 15 minutes

For Sauce

2 tablespoons butter 2 tablespoons yellow onion,

chopped

2 garlic cloves, minced 1 teaspoon fresh thyme,

chopped finely

1 1/3 cups homemade beef broth 2 tablespoons fresh lemon

juice

¾ cup fresh blueberries

For Steak

1 tablespoon butter 4 (6-ounce) grass-fed flank

steaks

Salt and ground black pepper, as required

- For sauce: in a pan, melt the butter over medium heat and sauté the

onion for about 2 minutes.

- Add the garlic and thyme and sauté for about 1 minute.
- Add the broth and bring to a gentle simmer.
- Reduce the heat to low and simmer for about 10 minutes.
- Meanwhile, for steak in a skillet, melt the butter over medium-high

heat and cook steaks with salt and black pepper for about 3-4

minutes per side.

- Transfer the steak into a bowl.
- Add the sauce in the skillet and stir to scrape up the

brown bits.

- Stir in the lemon juice, blueberries, salt and black pepper and cook

for about 1-2 minutes.

- Serve the steaks with the topping of sauce
- Meal Prep Tip: Transfer the steak with sauce into a large bowl and

set aside to cool completely. Divide the mixture into 4 containers

evenly. Cover the containers and refrigerate for up to 3-4 days.

Reheat in the microwave before serving.

One Serving: Net Carbs: 4.6g; Calories: 441; Total Fat: 23.4g; Sat. Fat:

11.5g; Protein: 49.5g; Carbs: 5.5g; Fiber: 0.9g; Sugar: 3.3g

Crab Salad

Serves: 4 / Preparation time: 15 minutes

1 pound jumbo lump crabmeat, picked over

1 celery stalk, peeled, and cut into 1/8-inch pieces

4 teaspoons fresh chives, minced 1 teaspoon fresh tarragon leaves, minced

1/3 cup mayonnaise 2 tablespoons sour cream

1 teaspoon fresh lemon juice ½ teaspoon Dijon mustard

Salt and ground black pepper, as required

- In a bowl, add the crabmeat, celery, chives and tarragon and toss to

coat well.

- In another bowl, add the mayonnaise, sour cream, lemon juice,

mustard, salt and black pepper and mix until well combined.

- Place the dressing into the bowl of the crabmeat mixture and gently,

stir to combine.

- Serve immediately.
- Meal Prep Tip: In 6 containers, divide salad and refrigerate for about

1 day.

One Serving: Net Carbs: 1.5g; Calories: 236; Total Fat: 16.7g; Sat. Fat:

2.8g; Protein: 14.5g; Carbs: 2.6g; Fiber: 0.1g; Sugar: 0.1g g

CPSIA information can be obtained
at www.ICGtesting.com
Printed in the USA
BVHW072320200421
605395BV00007B/1392

9 781802 327243